Gastric Sleeve Diet

Step By Step Guide For Planning What to Do and Eat Before and After Your Surgery

Bonus: FREE Report
Reveals The Secrets To Lose Weight

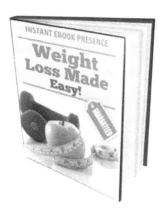

Weight loss doesn't happen from dieting only. Diets are short term solutions to shed extra weight. Diets do not work in the long term because people hate being on a diet (it's ok, you can admit that here). The only long term solution for permanent weight loss is to create new eating habits. This doesn't mean that chocolate will never pass your lips again, but it does mean looking after yourself and watching what you eat...

You can lose weight when you have the right reasons and motivation, and a part of this guide is to help you to find the motivation you need to change your weight...

Go To Get This Guid For FREE
http://www.sportsforsoul.com/weight-loss-2/

Table Of Contents:

Introduction

I want to thank you and congratulate you for downloading the book, *"Gastric Sleeve Diet Guide: Planning What to Do and Eat Before and After Your Surgery."* This book gives an overall, but detailed, view of the various aspects regarding the patient's experience with gastric sleeve surgery.

Gastric sleeve surgery is compared to gastric bypass surgery so that the reader can be confident that the gastric sleeve procedure is the right choice for them. Various risks associated with each procedure, though not likely, are discussed.

Proven steps and strategies on various things the gastric sleeve patient needs to do and eat before their surgery are discussed. Emphasis is made on how to find the correct surgeon for you. Many common questions that gastric sleeve patients have are answered in this book, including the subjects of stomach stretching and pain.

Common diets for the two-week period before the surgery and for the various time periods following the surgery are given, as well as the reasons the patient needs to stay on the surgeon's prescribed diet. Recipes are not included in this book.

Every effort was made to give the reader the information that he needs to plan a course to safely reach his or her weight loss goal through the use of the gastric sleeve procedure.

Thanks again for downloading this book. I hope you enjoy it!

Chapter 1: Be Sure About Your Procedure Choice

What Gastric Sleeve Surgery is

The other name for this procedure is *sleeve gastrectomy*. It is a *restrictive operation* that makes your stomach smaller so that you will feel fuller quicker and eat less food. This procedure involves the removal of more than half of your stomach. After your surgery, only a vertical tube that is about the size of a banana is left.

This surgery should be considered as a tool for weight loss rather than a quick fix because the patient will need to eat a healthy diet and exercise following the surgery. It is not cosmetic surgery where fat is removed. Only part of the stomach is removed.

History

United Healthcare (insurance) added sleeve gastrectomy to their list of surgeries that they cover for weight loss on January 1, 2010. Almost all other major health insurance companies began to cover this procedure during the next two years.

It is extremely difficult to get health insurance companies to approve new procedures, but gastric sleeve surgery was approved because there was evidence that the procedure brought about significant weight loss and the complication rates were low.

Additionally, surgeons were already doing the procedure on patients who were covered by insurance. This was an accomplishment because surgery on obese people is riskier than surgery on people of normal size.

The gastric sleeve procedure initially was the first of two surgeries that were normally done. Insurance companies paid for the first surgery and then paid for the second one a year or so later after weight was lost. However, it was discovered that the sleeve procedure was successful in getting people's weight off without the second surgery being done.

Sleeve patients lost as much weight as the gastric bypass patients did over time. The gastric sleeve procedure proved to be quicker, less complicated, and safer than the gastric bypass procedure, and the surgeons quickly started to prefer performing the sleeve operations.

Patients liked the results too because they just didn't experience hunger anymore. In fact, some of them had to remind themselves to eat.

Reasons for Gastric Sleeve Surgery

This surgery is done to help people to lose weight and to keep the extra weight off. This procedure is done when the patient is severely overweight and has been unable to lose weight through diet, exercise or medicine and where emotional eating was not the cause for the weight gain.

Even though the smaller stomach can eventually be stretched out to accommodate more food, this surgery encourages the patient to eat less food so that obesity won't remain a problem.

Candidates for this procedure have a body mass index that is 40 - 60 (or even higher) and/or they have a weight-related life-threatening or disabling problem and a body mass index of at least 35.

Studies show that obese people who undergo this surgery are less likely to die from cancer, diabetes and heart problems than obese people who never lose the weight.

The gastric sleeve procedure is less risky than a gastric bypass is because the small intestine is not divided and reconnected like it is in a bypass procedure. Major complications that require re-operation occur in less than 5% of gastric sleeve patients.

Even though the gastric sleeve surgery is now often the only gastric procedure that is performed on the patient, it is still sometimes done as part of a larger approach where this surgery is followed up with an intestinal rerouting procedure. The weight loss that occurs as a result of the first surgery often makes the second one unnecessary.

Sometimes a surgeon who goes into surgery planning to perform a gastric bypass procedure changes his mind during the operation in favor of performing a gastric sleeve procedure because of an enlarged liver or an extensive amount of scar tissue in the intestines that make a gastric bypass impossible.

Other reasons people get the gastric sleeve surgery include body severe comorbidities, Crohn's disease, advanced age, a need to surveil the stomach or to continue taking specific medications, or any combination of the above that increases risk for the patient if the bypass procedure were done.

To Get the Sleeve or a Bypass...That is the Question

Be sure that it is the gastric sleeve procedure that you want and not the gastric bypass procedure.

Even though it is the riskiest type of bariatric surgery, the gastric bypass procedure still accounts for about 80% of the bariatric procedures that are done in the United States. Laparoscopic adjustable gastric band and the gastric sleeve procedure make up the other 20%, perhaps because the sleeve is a relatively new procedure and not all surgeons know how to perform it.

If the sleeve procedure is done laparoscopically rather than by open surgery, it is sometimes referred to as a laparoscopic sleeve gastrectomy. The laparoscopic sleeve gastrectomy is a fairly new procedure, but it is growing in popularity.

Gastric bypass surgery - In the gastric bypass procedure, the intestines are bypassed. The shortened intestines give your body less time to absorb the calories. The stomach is also made smaller.

The power of this method is therefore twofold because the patient loses weight from a restricted size of their stomach (they eat less food) and from malabsorption of calories.

Additionally, eating junk food or eating too much food for the small capacity will make the person who has had this procedure very sick. You can read information about "dumping" below in the gastric bypass benefits section. Dumping undigested food into the small intestine makes the patient sick.

Gastric bypass surgery is recommended for people who have a body mass index that is over 45. The gastric bypass procedure makes the body lose 60 – 80% of the extra weight in just a year's time in and forces a change in eating habits.

Gastric sleeve surgery - Conversely, gastric sleeve patients only lose between 50 and 70 percent of it over twice the length of time - two years. However, patients who undergo this surgery do tend to catch up with the weight loss of the bypass procedure within three years and they appear better toned when they get there than bypass patients do because of losing the weight more gradually.

This surgery involves the removal of 70% of the stomach in the area where the hunger hormone is produced. Therefore, much of the weight-loss power of the gastric sleeve option is in the fact that the patient doesn't get very hungry.

Even though this surgery has been used as the first of two procedures that are done to obtain considerable weight loss, many surgeons find that many super-obese gastric sleeve patients lose a sufficient amount of weight following the gastric sleeve surgery to make the planned second surgery (to reroute the intestines) unnecessary.

Both the gastric bypass procedure and the gastric sleeve procedure can be done either laparoscopically or by open surgery, but laparoscopically is becoming ever more popular.

Laparoscopic Method – In this method, several small incisions are made in the abdomen, so it is much less invasive than the open method is. The surgery on the stomach is done using a camera to guide the surgeon and small instruments to perform the operation with. This method is becoming more and more popular.

Open Method – In open surgery, the surgeon makes a large incision, laying the patient open to be worked on in traditional fashion.

Both the gastric bypass and the gastric sleeve surgeries are permanent, so you need to be very sure about which procedure you want because you cannot reverse what is done in these two surgeries.

Factors to Consider – The decision to have a gastric sleeve surgery or a gastric bypass surgery depends on:

The gastric sleeve benefits over those of bypass

- Less complicated - The gastric sleeve procedure is less complicated than the bypass procedure is, so it is also less risky because the small intestine is not cut and then reconnected in this procedure as it is in the bypass procedure.

- Shorter operation time - The operation time for the gastric sleeve is shorter than the time it takes to do a bypass, which makes the sleeve a little safer.

- Works through hunger reduction - The gastric sleeve works through reducing hunger in the patient since 70% of the stomach area that produces the hunger hormone ghrelin is removed. Some patients have to remind themselves to eat for a half of a year after their surgery. The bypass procedure also reduces hunger a bit, but not as much as the sleeve procedure does.

- Slower rate of weight loss – It takes the body about 18 months to lose a massive amount of weight following a gastric sleeve procedure, which is slower than the loss that follows a bypass but faster than the lap band.

- Better appearance in the end - The slower pace of weight loss produces less saggy skin and fewer stretch marks than you would get with the super-fast weight loss that comes from the bypass procedure.

- Fewer vitamins required to be purchased for the remainder of life - You will need to buy fewer vitamins after this procedure than you will following the bypass surgery.

- Lower mortality rate - The mortality rate is lower from this procedure than it is from the bypass procedure, although it is below 1% for both procedures.

- Far less dumping episodes - The sleeve doesn't produce the dumping syndrome nearly as much as the bypass procedure does, so you won't get terribly sick should you eat something that is off of your diet. Sugar has time to digest. You may consider dumping to be a benefit of the bypass, however, since it prevents you from eating junk food for the rest of your life!

- No adjustments needed - Compared to the lap band, no adjustments are needed.

The <u>gastric bypass benefits</u> over those of the sleeve

- Long-established, well-known procedure - The bypass procedure has been around longer than the sleeve method and is considered "the gold standard." Laparoscopic surgeons have a lot of experience in the gastric bypass procedure.

- Few calories absorbed - Since much of the intestines are bypassed and the used part is short, you don't consume as many calories as you do if the full length of the intestines is used.

- Lowers GERD risk - The gastric bypass lowers your risk of acid reflux (GERD), so your surgeon will likely recommend you opt for the bypass if you have a history of acid reflux.

- Big weight loss immediately - Gastric bypass patients lose between 60 and 80 percent of their excess body weight during the first year following their surgery. This massive weight loss happens because of the unpleasant experience of the *dumping syndrome* that occurs whenever the patient eats or drinks sugary or fatty (junk) food and drink.

  The dumping syndrome is a condition where undigested sweet or fatty foods pass through the stomach and into the small intestine rapidly, causing nausea, vomiting, diarrhea, cramping, dizziness and fatigue.

Some people view this dumping aspect of the bypass procedure to be a   positive thing rather than a negative thing because it forces them to eat better.

Dumping usually happens just 15 to 30 minutes after eating junk food. Late dumping happens after three hours and just makes people sweat and feel weak and dizzy. Some people experience both types of dumping.

Why we are not discussing lap band

Many surgeons who have a good amount of experience in lap band, sleeve gastrectomy and in gastric bypass surgeries have found that many of the people who get the lap band don't end up losing weight because the lap band patients often don't dedicate themselves to changing their diet and to exercising. *While patients who have the other procedures done must also change their lifestyle, the failure rate is much higher in lap band patients.*

Surgeons want their patients to succeed for both the patients' sake and for their own reputation. Patients who lose a lot of weight will likely refer other people to the surgeon. Surgeons cannot always determine which people will follow a new diet and exercise regimen and which ones will not.

Additionally, the lap band is a hassle for both the patient and the surgeon after a lap band is put into the patient's body because the patient must go back to the surgeon several times per year for the rest of the patient's life to get the band fill levels checked. With a sleeve or a bypass operation, no foreign object has been inserted, and the patient is done with the surgeon after a few check-ups.

How long the surgery would be for gastric sleeve versus gastric bypass

It is always risky to be under anesthesia. It is even higher for obese people to be under anesthesia. High cholesterol and high blood pressure increase the risks even more. While procedural time is a minor factor in making your decision, but it should still be considered when the risk is highest.

The average surgery time for a *gastric sleeve* operation is only 1 hour and 40 minutes, but the average surgery time for a *gastric bypass* operation is 2 hours and almost 45 minutes.

How fast I will lose weight after gastric sleeve versus gastric bypass

As previously stated, weight loss from *gastric bypass* is greater from the start in comparison to *gastric sleeve* surgery, however, weight loss after the gastric sleeve begins to catch up within three years after the surgery. The slower weight loss time following the gastric sleeve surgery also produces less saggy skin and fewer stretch marks. Still, some people prefer to get skinny quickly.

Body mass index affects the speed of weight loss too because the higher the patient's initial body mass index, the more weight they lose, no matter which method is used.

Chapter 2: Compare Sleeve Complications to Bypass Complications

There are several more complications associated with the gastric bypass procedure than with the gastric sleeve procedure. You should take a look at what the complications are with each option, especially if you are still not sure which procedure to have.

	Sleeve	Bypass
Gastroesophageal Reflux Disease (GERD)	X	
Staple line failure (then infection, abscess...)	X	
Stricture (chronic)	X	
Stricture (acute)	X	X
Nutritional deficiencies	X	X
Gallstones	X	X
Venous thromboembolism	X	X
Death	X	X
Nausea		X
Dehydration		X
Indigestion		X
Reactive hypoglycemia		X
Incisional hernia		X
Wound infection		X
Marginal ulcers		X
Stomal stenosis (Stricture)		X
Anastomotic leaks		X
Hemorrhage		X

Gastroesophageal Reflux Disease (GERD)

With risk as high as 47%, GERD is a very common complication that *gastric sleeve* patients experience. It starts off with occasional episodes of gastroesophageal reflux and heartburn. As time goes on, the esophagus structure changes and the patient gets inflammation of the esophagus for which the patient takes proton pump inhibitors.

Staple Line Failure

This complication is one that surgeons try to prevent. Special attention is given to putting staples into the stomach where the stomach is reattached to itself.

In a staple line failure, food and drink get through this area, getting into the abdominal cavity. When food and drink get into the abdominal cavity, an infection called peritonitis sets in, which can become life-threatening.

Symptoms include a rapid heart rate, chills, fever, nausea, vomiting, swelling of the abdomen, rapid breathing, and/or severe pain.

If it happens within a week following the gastric sleeve surgery, a laparoscopy may be attempted to locate and repair the leaking area. If the leak happens after a week, the area is drained and washed out, etc. The risk of line failure is 2.4%.

Stricture (chronic)

Chronic stricture is a complication that is associated with *gastric sleeve* surgery, and it is the narrowing of the stomach outlet area at the place where it is attached surgically to the small bowel. With this condition, the patient has trouble eating solid food, has increased saliva and/or mucus, and also has reflux symptoms.

Stricture can happen after a month or two following your surgery. Sometimes it resolves itself in time. If it doesn't resolve itself, the treatment options depend on how long the narrow portion is. Endoscopic dilation is used when the narrowed portion is short. If the narrowed portion is long, repeated endoscopic dilation may be performed so as to fix the problem. If repeated dilation fails, the patient may then get the gastric bypass done.

Stricture (acute)

This condition more commonly follows *gastric bypass* surgery, but it sometimes happens to *gastric sleeve* patients.

Acute stricture is an acute narrowing of the stomach outlet area at the place where it is attached surgically to the small bowel. With this condition, the opening is so narrow that the patient even has trouble getting liquids through. The patient also experiences increased saliva and/or mucus, and reflux symptoms.

This can happen after a month or two following your surgery. Treatment involves replacing food and liquids with IV fluids and endoscopic dilation. There is a 3.5% risk for getting either a chronic or acute stricture following (usually bypass) surgery.

Nutritional deficiencies

Malnutrition is possible in both *gastric sleeve* and *gastric bypass* patients, especially if the supplements are not taken. Deficiencies for which you will need to compensate for with supplements for the rest of your life following your gastric surgery include the following:

Iron – Iron is needed for red blood cell production, for liver parenchymal cells, and for the reticuloendothelial system. Iron deficiency anemia will occur if supplements are not taken, especially in women of reproductive age who are menstruating.

Calcium and *Vitamin D* – A reduction in calcium, vitamin D and exercise will eventually result in bone resorption and osteoporosis.

Vitamin B12 – Deficiency in B12 results in emotional changes (depression, psychosis, and depression), decreased thinking capabilities, poor muscle function, changes in reflexes, low red blood cells, decreased fertility, reduced heart function, inflammation of the tongue and decreased taste.

Folate – This B vitamin makes and repairs DNA and produces red blood cells. A deficiency of this vitamin results in anemia, which deprives your tissues of oxygen and then affects their function. Birth defects are sometimes caused by folate deficiency during pregnancy. Folate deficiency symptoms include growth problems, tongue swelling, mouth sores, gray hair and fatigue. Folate deficiency leads to anemia, which has the symptoms of irritability, shortness of breath, pale skin, lethargy, weakness and persistent fatigue. Fortified cereals, fruits and vegetables contain folate.

Vitamin A – Night blindness is caused by lack of vitamin A in the diet, as is a diminished ability to fight off infections and maternal mortality.

Vitamin E – Deficiency in vitamin E causes neurological and neuromuscular problems, anemia, retinopathy and impairment of the immune response.

Vitamin K – A lack of vitamin K can result in massive uncontrolled bleeding, bleeding at the surgical sites, stomach pains, cartilage calcification, and malformation of developing bone. This vitamin in used by the liver to create enzymes needed for coagulation of the blood.

Selenium – Insufficient selenium results in muscle wasting, muscle myopathy, arrhythmia, cardiomyopathy, reduced thyroid, and immunity function. Loss of hair and skin pigment can also occur, along with encephalopathy and white nail beds. Absorption of selenium is helped along with vitamins C and E.

Protein – Protein prevents hair loss, sickness, flaky dermatitis, and fluid retention in the ankles and feet. Protein keeps bones, skin, nails, and hair healthy. Malabsorption can also lead to kidney oxalate stones and lactic acidosis.

Most importantly for the gastric sleeve patient, protein aids in proper wound healing and promotes weight loss. Protein helps with weight loss several ways.

- It satisfies and therefore discourages a dieter from eating extra calories due to hunger. Protein helps a person to feel full, strong and energized because protein takes longer to digest than carbs and some other foods do.

- The presence of protein ensures that it is fat and not metabolism-boosting muscle the body uses for fuel. If a person does not get enough protein, the body breaks down muscles to get what it needs. A person needs at least 50 and 60 grams of protein daily to prevent the loss of body muscle mass.

- Additionally, protein food requires the body to burn more calories to process than other kinds of food do.

Because the stomach of a gastric sleeve patient is small, protein needs to be consumed first so that the patient doesn't become too full to eat or drink protein. Both plant and animal sources of protein are needed in the food that is eaten.

Smoothies and shakes made with protein powders and other proper ingredients are useful for delivering a lot of protein in a small amount of drink, which is especially helpful in the first few weeks following a gastric sleeve surgery. Some people also take liquid protein supplements.

Men need between 70 and 90 grams of protein and women need between 60 and 80 grams of protein daily. The risk of protein deficiency in the gastric sleeve patient is about 12%.

Gallstones

Gallstones affect both *gastric sleeve* and *gastric bypass* patients. The risk of getting this complication is as high as 23% in people who lose a large amount of weight, but they are only a problem if they block the opening to the gallbladder. Bile salts prevent them from forming in the bile ducts or in the gallbladder, but the surgery causes malabsorption or the bile salts. If you have an attack, you will need to have surgery for it because it won't go away on its own.

Venous Thromboembolism

This condition is much more common in *gastric bypass* patients than in *gastric sleeve* patients, but it does occur following either procedure. The risk for this problem, whether a deep vein thrombosis or a pulmonary embolism, is less than one percent in gastric sleeve patients.

Death

It is possible to die from complications that arise following *either* one of these two gastric procedures.

Nausea

Nausea commonly follows gastric bypass surgery, but not gastric sleeve surgery. This condition is helped by following the diet that the patient's doctor or nutritionist recommends following the operation. A large amount of IV fluid will also help to alleviate nausea. The risk for this complication is 70% for the bypass patient.

Dehydration

Depletion of fluids is common in *gastric bypass* patients, but not in gastric sleeve patients. The risk is as high as 65% for bypass patients. Dehydration is resolved by drinking two liters of fluids per day. Vomiting and further dehydration occur if the bypass patient does not drink enough water. An IV line may be necessary if the dehydration gets bad enough.

Indigestion

Indigestion is a complication of *gastric bypass* surgery (but not gastric sleeve surgery), affecting 60% of patients. It can be defined as digestion difficulty that is accompanied by discomfort or burning in the upper abdomen.

It is helped by the avoidance of greasy food or possibly drinking only liquids for a while. H2 blockers and antacids are used if dietary changes don't solve the problem.

Reactive Hypoglycemia

Reactive hypoglycemia sometimes follows *gastric bypass* surgery, but not gastric sleeve surgery, and it happens between 45 and 60 minutes after a patient who has a low blood sugar eats a high-carbohydrate meal. It also often occurs because of the excessive "dumping" of undigested food into the small intestines that happens in bypass patients.

The person gets lightheaded, sweaty and their heart rate increases because of the imbalance between insulin and blood sugar in the bloodstream. Insulin that remains after blood sugar is used causes low blood sugar.

To resolve the situation, the patient needs to drink two ounces of skim milk or a few ounces of diluted juice. This condition can be prevented by eating proteins first and avoiding the consumption of sugar. Additionally, medications are sometimes prescribed to manage the condition. Part of the pancreas is removed in extreme situations so as to manage this condition. The risk for reactive hypoglycemia is only 1%.

Incisional Hernia

An Incisional hernia sometimes follows *gastric bypass* surgery, but not usually gastric sleeve surgery. An incisional hernia is an opening that forms when an internal body part or organ comes out through a surgical incision because of the incision not healing correctly. This is a dangerous condition because the intestine becomes obstructed.

This kind of hernia occurs in 20% of patients who have an open surgical procedure and in only 0.2% of patients who have laparoscopic procedures, and they show up several months after the procedure.

Wound Infection

Wound infection sometimes follows *gastric bypass* surgery, but not gastric sleeve surgery. Bacteria are released from the bowel while the stomach is being operated on, infecting the incisions. Sometimes the inside of the abdomen is what get infected. Additionally, kidney and bladder infections can occur.

Physical activity, respiratory therapy, and, of course, antibiotics after surgery can lower the risk of infection. The risk level of wound infection is 12%, with the vast majority occurring in patients who underwent open surgery instead of laparoscopic surgery.

Marginal Ulcers

Marginal ulcers sometimes follow *gastric bypass* surgery, but not gastric sleeve surgery. A new stomach pouch is created when a person undergoes gastric bypass surgery and this kind of ulcer most commonly forms in the new pouch. A burning pain in the stomach is common to ulcer sufferers.

Proper dietary habits and the avoidance of smoking and NSAIDs help the bypass patient to avoid getting marginal ulcers. Endoscopy can be performed to confirm their presence, but their treatment is usually just antacids. The risk factor for getting this is 12%.

Stomal Stenosis (Stricture)

Stomal stenosis sometimes follows *gastric bypass* surgery, but not usually following gastric sleeve surgery, although it can. It results from the buildup of scar tissue. This condition involves inflammation or blockage of the opening to or from the stomach, which prevents food from entering the stomach or intestines. It can be chronic or acute.

Symptoms include food intolerance, nausea, vomiting, and dysphagia. It is treated by fasting and hydration by IV. A second plan is an endoscopic dilation. The risk for this is 8%.

Anastomotic Leaks

Anastomotic leaks sometimes follow *gastric bypass* surgery, but not gastric sleeve surgery. This leak happens during surgery and is when digestive contents get into the abdomen when a connection is being made. It can be fixed if found quickly enough but can become infected if it is not found. A dye is used to see if the connection is secure. The risk factor is 5%.

Hemorrhage (bleeding)

Hemorrhages sometimes follow *gastric bypass* surgery, but not gastric sleeve surgery. Bleeding that sometimes follows bypass surgery include vomiting blood (hematemesis) or blood in the stools (melena stools). The risk for one of these is 3.2%.

Chapter 3: Ten Crucial Steps to Take Before Your Gastric Sleeve Surgery

Okay, now that you are sure about your decision to get the sleeve gastrectomy, there are some things that you need to think about and to do before you go in for your surgery. Here are some steps that you need to take.

Step One: Find out whether or not you qualify for a gastric sleeve surgery.

If you want to have weight loss surgery in the United States, there are some particular requirements that the National Institute of Health (NIH) says that you need to meet. You need to 1) be over 18 years old, and 2) have a body mass index of 40 or more or have a body mass index of 35 and one or more comorbid conditions.

The body mass index is a measurement of height over weight. Comorbid conditions are diseases that result from being overweight or are strongly related to being overweight. These conditions include, but are not limited to, soft tissue infections, venous stasis disease, type 2 diabetes, high cholesterol, high blood pressure, sleep apnea and arthritis.

Step Two: Find out whether or not your insurance will cover weight loss surgery.

Although you must be morbidly obese, being morbidly obese does not mean your insurance will cover the surgery. That is a separate thing you need to pursue. The insurance companies require what the NHI requires and often more.

The aforementioned conditions are usually covered by insurance. Sometimes an insurance company will also cover acid reflux disease, psychosocial stress resulting from obesity, stroke or risk of stroke, depression, gallbladder disease, fatty liver syndrome and/or congestive heart failure.

Visit ObesityCoverage.com to use their insurance checker tool.

Step Three: Find two potential surgeons.

To find a couple of potential surgeons, you will have to research, get onto some online forums, and possibly ask around.

Step Four: Attend a seminar.

Once you have a couple of candidates for a good surgeon, you need to learn some things from them. Surgeons usually have a way that you can register on their website to attend an in-person seminar. Sometimes an online seminar is available too.

Step Five: Set up a consultation with one or more of the surgeons you selected.

After you learn general things from the seminar's information, you'll likely have some questions for the surgeon that you select to perform your operation. Set up and attend a consultation with the surgeon. Have those questions ready to ask him. See the Frequently Asked Questions information for what questions you might want to ask.

Step Six: Obtain a Letter of Medical Necessity from your primary care physician.

Get your regular doctor to write for you a Letter of Medical Necessity to clear you for surgery.

Step Seven: Obtain insurance pre-approval for you to have the operation.

The surgeon's office will turn in your paperwork for you, but you need to call them from time to time to keep on top of where things stand.

Step Eight: Get the psychiatric tests and lab work done and obtain a medically supervised diet.

The surgeon will refer you to local providers who will administer the various tests.

Step Nine: Choose a surgery date. Make plans to be off of work for a while.

After you are approved for the surgery, choose a surgery date. Make plans to be off of work for at least two weeks. You won't want to lift heavy things, so judge the situation for yourself and allow yourself adequate time to heal properly.

Step Ten: Keep yourself focused, motivated and engaged in the process.

Get yourself involved in your own weight loss project, doing whatever that means for you. For example, you could study the experiences of other people and gather recipes for protein shakes, pureed food, and soft food that you think you might enjoy and try some of the recipes. Shop for food. Pre-make and freeze shakes (minus the ice) and other foods. You could get your helpers lined up, get ahead of the household laundry, cleaning, and other chores, including buying your vitamins and medicines, etc. Get excited and move things forward!

Chapter 4: Choosing the Right Surgeon for You

How do I choose a bariatric surgeon?

A local surgeon may be important to you because you will have to go see your surgeon several times before the surgery and several times after the surgery. Isolation often results in failed weight loss.

If the surgeon is not local, flying for the many visits you'll need to take is not a good option. Ask various surgeons how they accommodate out-of-town patients in things like recommendations for post-op visits, hotels, and whether or not you can check in without having to travel.

Research surgeons and their support staff through various methods. You can read about various surgeons online. You can read what others have to say in the various online support groups. You can ask acquaintances about surgeons they may have heard of or had experience with.

You want your surgeon to have credentials, so you will want him to:
- Be fellowship-trained as a bariatric surgeon
- Be board-certified in general surgery
- Participate in groups like the American Society of Metabolic and Bariatric Surgeons
- Participate in continuing education in bariatric surgery
- Have the support staff and adequate aftercare resources for you
- Have adequate experience performing gastric sleeve operations in the method you have chosen (laparoscopic or open)

You may want to meet some of his previous patients. You want to be able to trust the surgeon to meet your needs, listen to your concerns, answer your questions, give excellent care after the surgery, and offer various kinds of support

You may want to have your gastric sleeve surgery performed at a specialized hospital, one that is a Center of Excellence in bariatric surgery. Center of Excellence is a designation that says that the facility has:

- Has achieved excellence in their surgeries
- Has performed a specific minimum number of bariatric procedures during the prior year
- Staff that has taken extra training in weight loss surgery
- A bariatric coordinator who ensures that things run smoothly, often serving as the patient's main point of contact

You can find a Center of Excellence on the MBSAQIP (Metabolic and Bariatric Surgery Accreditation and Quality Improvement Program) website. Then you can choose from among the surgeons who practice there and make your surgeon selection that way. Don't rule out regular hospitals, however.

What do I ask the bariatric surgeon?

Once you have narrowed down a few surgeons and a hospital or two, you want a consultation with one or more surgeons, ask the questions listed below and any other questions you need answers to. Then select a surgeon.

1.) *Ask him about his surgery experience.* Ten years of experience is a respectable amount of experience with surgery and assures that he can handle any difficulties.

Even though having a lot of experience is desirable, the experience is not the same thing as skill. Some younger surgeons, even ones just coming out of a quality training program, can do a good job. They are likely in a two-year fellowship program where they specialize in a type of surgery.

Remember that the gastric sleeve procedure is one of the newer gastric procedures, so nobody has long-term experience with it. Fortunately, the gastric sleeve surgery is simpler and less risky than the bypass surgery procedure is and quickly gained the confidence of health insurance companies.

You also want to know specifically what his experience is with the particular method he plans to use on you, i.e. laparoscopic surgery vs. open surgery.

2.) *Ask the surgeon what resources he offers before and after the surgery.* Your weight loss success depends on more than just having had the operation. You will need to change how you eat and start to exercise too, so it would be useful to you if the surgeon has some resources available that would support you while you go on the weight loss journey. You need a good surgeon who also has a good bariatric coordinator and dietitian.

A dietician who listens to you and can work out a plan for you that is tailored to your situation would be a great resource. Some surgeons offer online support groups, weekly in-person support groups and/or Facebook support groups that discuss various subjects relating to life after bariatric surgery. Smartphone apps that keep you connected are also offered by some surgeons.

3.) Ask the surgeon which procedures he performs. Not all surgeons offer all procedures or know how to do all of them. Ask why they don't offer the one(s) they don't offer. If they push for one kind of surgery, they may have some sort of self-interest involved and you may benefit more from a different surgeon.

You likely have an enlarged liver. If it is too large, its size would prevent the sleeve procedure from being done laparoscopically because the doctor would not be able to push the liver far enough to the side to access your stomach. If the surgeon also knows how to do a sleeve gastrectomy using the open method or if he knows how to do the bypass surgery, there are more options available to get the job done while you are under anesthesia. You wouldn't want him to just sew you up having done nothing for lack of knowledge.

4.) Ask the surgeon which procedure he recommends for you. A good surgeon would know that one procedure is not the best fit for every person. A good surgeon will want to find out more about you before he answers the question. He'll need to know what you eat, how much you exercise, what your risk tolerances are, etc. If you do emotional eating or binge eating, he may suggest you get the bypass surgery instead of the sleeve procedure because the bypass procedure will force you to change your eating habits.

And actually, he would try to present you with the risks and the benefits associated with each procedure as they relate to you and let you decide.

Talk to your surgeon about your goals and about your fears. Be confident that you are making the right procedure choice and surgeon choice before you have a procedure done.

If he rushes through your consultation, your future experiences with him will likely also be rushed. You will see the surgeon several times before your surgery and a few times during the following year after your surgery, so you need to be able to benefit from your visits with him.

5.) *Ask the surgeon what his complication rates are.* These are complications that occur during or around the time of the operation. They do not include minor postoperative complications.

The national averages for complications during the various surgeries are 3.6% for gastric bypass, **2.2% for a gastric sleeve**, and just 0.9% for lap band procedures, so you want this surgeon's complication rate to be at or below the national average of 2.2% for gastric sleeve surgeries. Hopefully, he has enough surgeries under his belt (at least 100) so that it would be possible to get a truly representative percentage.

6.) *Ask the surgeon why you should select him to do the operation.* This will be an unusual question for a surgeon to receive, but if he can answer it with something about how he loves his job and will be supportive of you on your journey, you may be more comfortable with him than if he just brags about his skills.

Chapter 5: More Questions to Ask before Surgery

How much weight can I expect to lose?

You need to know how much weight you should expect to lose after the surgery. Do the calculations and you will know. You will lose somewhere around 60% of the extra weight over two years, with likely the majority of it coming off in the first year.

Long-term weight loss, however, is more dependent on what you eat, how much you exercise, etc. than on which one of the procedures you choose. It is possible to gain all of the weight back.

Will my stomach stretch after surgery?

It can stretch, but it depends on how much you normally feed it. For an occasional large meal, your stomach can stretch to accommodate it and then get back to its smaller size. However, if you continue to give it large meals (or meals too large for the size your stomach will be), then it can and will stretch and not get back to its smaller size. If you stretch it back out, you eat more food. When you eat more food, you gain weight.

People often become fat because their hunger and full signals are actually broken. It would be best to monitor how much food you eat. Even an occasional small sweet is better than an excessively large amount of quality food because you are not stretching your stomach.

Can I still drink alcohol after my gastric sleeve surgery?

Yes, you can have alcohol after your surgery, but it will make you drunker much faster than before you have your surgery because of having a smaller stomach that holds less food. It would be advisable to just give up alcohol.

While you can have wine or something after your surgery, you need to be very aware that one or two glasses of wine for you would have the same effect as six or seven glasses of wine would have on a person who has a normal-sized stomach. If you do that regularly, you become an alcoholic.

In fact, studies show that many people who have no history of alcohol abuse easily become alcoholics and get charged with DWIs from about two years after having a gastric sleeve surgery onward because they drink the same amount of alcohol they did before their surgery, not realizing the effect alcohol has on them after their stomach has become small.

Let your family know this if you drink at all so they can help you keep your alcohol consumption under control.

You also need to remember that alcohol is a carbohydrate as well as something that can make you drunk. As a carbohydrate, it has no nutritional benefit, and too much of it can cause you to gain weight. 'Too much" for a person with a small stomach is not very much.

Alcohol is also toxic to your body and will negatively affect your liver much faster than you would imagine it would. You will need to keep all of this information in mind if you must drink.

Besides sensitivities to alcohol, what other sensitivities might I expect as a result of having a smaller stomach?

You will be more sensitive to all carbohydrates and proteins consumed, as well as to the vitamins and minerals that you ingest.

In addition to food and drink, you will also be more sensitive to things that you smell. Chemicals and other odors may create responses that you did not have before you had your gastric surgery.

What can I expect in the way bowel movements after gastric sleeve surgery?

While you are on the liquid and pureed diets, the bowels won't have trouble, although pain medication can lead to some constipation. Follow the guidelines you will be given and you should be okay during those phases.

After you start to consume regular food, you can expect some changes in your bowel movements. Be prepared for more gas, occasional cramping, different smells than you are used to, and likely some constipation if you are not careful to include fiber and liquid in the diet.

After your gastric sleeve surgery, your metabolism will have slowed down due to consuming few calories. The combination of regular food, a slowed metabolism, and the effects of pain medication can create stools that are hard to pass. Of all times to not force things, after surgery is definitely not the time to force things.

Fluids and fiber in your diet should help to prevent a potential constipation problem. If you have ongoing problems with constipation, despite your efforts to avoid having a constipation problem, talk to your surgeon about it.

How much pain will I experience?

This question is hard to answer because of the different ways that people rate pain. Open surgery is quite painful and it also requires a longer hospital stay than does laparoscopic surgery.

The site of incision is where the pain comes from, which is the reason that laparoscopic surgery causes far less pain than open surgery does. If you follow the diet guidelines before surgery and get your liver smaller so that the surgeon can move it out of the way, your surgeon will be able to perform the much less painful laparoscopic procedure on you. Following those diet instructions helps both of you!

The upper left quadrant, which is under your rib cage, is the site where most of the pain comes from. The incision there is widened and stretched to get the part of the stomach that is being removed out. Muscle fibers tear in that area and bruising results. Even so, pain can be managed with pain medications for the first few days.

Surgery Day – You will wake up groggy and you won't have much pain at first because of the pain medication you were administered. You will feel general soreness wherever incisions were made. You may also be a little nauseated from the anesthesia at first.

Your surgeon may actually want you to get up and walk on this day to reduce the pain that the CO_2 caused during the surgery. It will be difficult to get out of the bed on this day because you will be sore. The rest of the day, you will be on your back with the bed slightly inclined upward.

Day One – You will notice the pain much more on this day because the anesthesia will have worn off. You will have pain medication, but you will be moving around a bit more on this day. They will have you use the IV pain medication less and use oral ones more. If you had your surgery laparoscopically, the pain will be bearable.

Your throat will still be sore, dry and swollen from the tube that was put down it while you were under anesthesia, but drinking a little water should help.

You will be rolled by wheelchair to Radiology for your swallow test. Your doctor will ask you about your pain level, remove your catheter, and make sure you are able to get up onto your feet. He'll also answer questions then. He will discharge you if you had your procedure done laparoscopically.

Day Two and Three – Your pain is still bearable if you had the laparoscopic procedure done. Days three through six will be your most painful days because you will be on your feet more often and turning your trunk to the side more than when you were in the hospital, but your doctor should have given you instructions for pain management for this period. Let your surgeon know if your pain is unbearable.

Week One – After a few days, life can be more normal, although pain can flare up any time you stand up from a seated position, twist your torso, or bend over for the next several weeks. All of that will go away in time, though.

Most people are still in too much pain to return to work during this week, though the pain is not severe. Getting into and out of a car and running errands will cause the most pain. Some people are too tired to return to work too.

Week Two to Month Three – You should not have much pain at all by the second month after surgery. You are likely off of pain medication. Contact your doctor if you are in nagging pain after two months.

Month Three to Six and Beyond – You should not notice pain hardly ever by this point. If you do, talk to the doctor. Gastric sleeve patients who have gone through the whole process and got the weight off say that the pain was worth it in the end.

What exactly is stomach stapling?

The stomach is literally stapled back together with a surgical staple gun when the surgeon performs either a gastric sleeve procedure or a gastric bypass.

The staples close in the shape of a "B" to both compress enough to not allow bleeding while also allowing the blood to flow through the holes of the B. Tissue can heal properly using this type of staple. Loading the wrong staple size for the thickness of tissue can cause leaks, however.

What happens to the staples?

The staples will stay in you forever because they are made of titanium. Even if they move from their original position, they won't cause problems. Additionally, they are not magnetic and will not set off any x-ray machines at airports or other places.

Am I ready to make changes?

You need to decide inside yourself that you like yourself and want to treat yourself good. Remember who you were before you got fat (if it hasn't been a lifetime thing). What made you, you? Remember how good you looked in normal sized clothes and how your appearance gave you some self-confidence and mobility to do more things.

Get a vision of the new you in your mind and focus on it frequently. Decide in your mind that from now on you will change your eating habits and also do more exercise. The surgery is just a tool to help you in your journey, but you only lose weight and keep it off through your own efforts to change your lifestyle.

What does gastric sleeve surgery cost?

There are costs associated with the surgery both before the surgery and after the surgery. Some of the after-surgery costs will remain for the rest of your life.

The nutritionist consultation price is negotiated before your visit. Consultations with a nutritionist range between $50.00 and $100.00 per visit, and you pay for them out of pocket.

Of course, you will buy the food, protein powders, clothing for various sizes, etc., before your surgery. If you don't have a blender, you'll likely need to buy one.

The price of gastric sleeve surgery itself is typically much less than the cost of a gastric bypass but slightly more than a gastric band surgery. Costs vary by state. Generally speaking, the procedure tends to be cheaper in the southern half of the United States than it is in the northern half. Fortunately, the costs have been coming down due to increased competition and demand for the surgery.

Costs for gastric sleeve surgery range *between $9,600 and $26,000 in the United States.* The cost for the procedure is most often quoted to be around $14,900, but *$16,800 is about the average price for it.*

These figures represent what it would cost you to pay for the procedure yourself. Insurance companies are charged more than this, however.

After your surgery, your follow-up visits with your surgeon are free. However, if you have complications, it will cost a lot of money to treat the complications.

Complications will be covered by insurance if the surgery was covered by insurance. They will be paid for by you if you paid for the surgery out of pocket. Wound site infections, which are caused by the surgeon, are usually paid for by the surgery center or hospital.

After your surgery, your new lifestyle will cost you some extra money in the following ways:

Quality food - Even though your stomach will be smaller, food will be more expensive because you will be eating better quality food.

Gym membership - You may get a gym membership.

Supplements – If you spend money on nothing else, you will need to spend money on supplements for the rest of your life so that you can function because you will be missing much of your stomach and will therefore not be able to absorb sufficient nutrients. Quality protein supplements alone can cost you more than $50.00 per month.

Clothing - You will have to keep buying new clothes as you keep losing weight if you don't have much of your old clothes or didn't buy some before your surgery. You may want to buy things at Goodwill or at yard sales until you reach your goal and plateau out.

Cosmetic surgery - You may have cosmetic surgery done to remove excess skin that may droop from your body. You can save up for that expense.

What do I need to do at home before my surgery?

Change your diet early – You need to start the protein liquid diet one or two weeks before you have your surgery. This is done to shrink your liver, and that will make the surgery safer for you.

Make out a different kind of grocery list – You need to have a lot of protein both before and after your surgery, so you will need to get familiar with some protein smoothie and shake recipes. They are made with protein powders which come in various flavors. You will need clear liquids before you can have the shakes and smoothies, so you'll need to also have broth, unsweetened juices, etc., on your shopping list and in your home.

Buy yourself some clothes (or dig out old ones) – Right after your surgery, you will want loose-fitting clothes and slippers. Then you will need to fit into various sizes of clothes as you lose weight while you also heal.

Stop smoking – Your surgeon will not perform the surgery if your body does not test as being smoke-free. That is because you will not recover as well as you would if you didn't have that in your system.

Pack your hospital bag – You will need to stay in the hospital only one night, so pack whatever you need to make yourself both comfortable and entertained.

Prepare your support group – After your surgery, you will need to have friends and family lined up to prepare and bring you your meals, pick up your prescription medications, help you with minor grooming, etc. They will need to be educated as to what your surgery entailed and what your limitations will be and for how long. Get people committed in helping you during certain days and times to do specific chores, etc., before surgery day.

Get your insurance or money lined up ahead of time – Refer to the insurance information under the steps given in this book and/or review the cost in the FAQ section above.

Get caught up with household chores, even pre-making your protein drinks – After your surgery, you won't want to or be able to do a lot of the things that you normally do for a while, so get ahead of the laundry, the housekeeping, the grocery shopping, clothes shopping, and anything else that you normally do that can be done ahead of time.

While you will (hopefully) have some helpers lined up, it would be helpful to everybody, including yourself, if you had most of the work done ahead of time and utilize your volunteers for things that you can't do ahead of time and would need help with right after surgery.

You will want a lot of smoothies and shakes because they pack a lot of protein in a small amount. You will likely be able to get around in the kitchen at this point, but you won't feel like doing projects, and smoothies and shakes call for fresh ingredients.

Fresh ingredients don't stay fresh for long, and you likely won't feel like driving, shopping and messing around a lot in the kitchen yet. Your helpers most likely will not want to shop for fresh ingredients, follow a recipe, cut and blend things either. That would make them feel imposed upon and regretful they volunteered to help you, so you really need to make smoothies and shakes ahead of time!

Make the smoothies and shakes up, minus the ice the recipes may call for, and pour them into ice cube trays for easy access and measurement into two ounces per cube. You could transfer the frozen smoothie or shake cubes to a container and label the container.

You won't be consuming much of anything for a while. Frozen cubed smoothies and shakes would allow small amounts of your pre-made, frozen smoothies and shakes to be easily accessed. When it is time for you to drink some, you or your helper can take out a couple of cubes and some ice shavings, blend them and pour the drink into your medicine (it has measurements) cup or whatever.

Get the facts – Do your homework and the steps mentioned. Once you have researched everything and talked to the surgeon of your choice, you will feel much more confident when you have your surgery.

Study the proteins – You will need to consume a lot of protein before and after your surgery, so explore and experiment with various sources of protein. Know what they are.

What do I need to take to the hospital?

It is totally up to you what you take to the hospital, but in general, you will want what makes you comfortable and keeps you entertained.

You may want lotion, lip balm, and grooming items. You may want your favorite pillow and/or pillowcase. Things that will make you comfortable clothes-wise may include house slippers for the hospital stay and loose-fitting clothes and slip-on shoes for that trip home.

You may want your electronic gadgets for keeping your family up to date on your progress using social media. You may want to read ebooks or surf the web. You may just want a good physical book or a stack of magazines for your entertainment in addition to the television that you will likely have in your room.

Chapter 6: Your Pre-Operation Diet

If you think that you can binge eat right up until operation day, you are wrong. Not only will you have to have stopped smoking about a month before operation day (to assure better healing), but you will need to have followed a strict diet for a couple of weeks. It is important for you to cooperate with the surgeon by following this diet before the surgery.

Since you are obese, there is a high likelihood that your liver is also full of fat. To access your stomach laparoscopically, the surgeon needs to be able to move your liver to the side. If it is still a fatty liver that he finds during your operation, moving it aside wouldn't make any difference to his inability to access your stomach laparoscopically.

The surgeon will likely cancel the operation or do your operation the open surgery method if you didn't follow instructions to shrink your liver's size through this two-week diet.

If the doctor can do your surgery laparoscopically, he can decrease the risk of complications during your surgery, the surgery will be performed quicker and easier, and you will experience significantly less pain than you would if you force the surgeon to perform the operation in the open surgery method.

The Requirements

Typically, you will be required to change your eating habits as follows:

- Increase protein consumption through lean meats, protein powders, etc.

- Lower your carbohydrate consumption by avoiding bread, pasta, cereal, rice, etc.

- Eliminate sugar, including candy, desserts, juices, soda, etc.

Two Weeks before your Surgery - Sample Pre-Operation Menu

A sample daily two-week, the pre-operation menu looks like the following:

Breakfast

Protein shake (even just one of the commercially made ones) that does not contain any sort of sugar

Lunch

     Lean meat plus vegetables

Dinner

     Lean meat plus vegetables

Snacks

     Low-carb, healthy options, such as nuts, berries, veggies, small salad with an oil and vinegar dressing

Fluids

     Drink lots of fluids that are sugar-free and low in calories

Two Days before Your Surgery – More Limitations

You will need to do the following for the two days before your surgery:

- Omit carbonated beverages

- Omit caffeine

- Go on a diet of clear liquids. Clear food consists of things like broth, sugar-free popsicles, sugar-free Jell-O, and water. You may get one protein shake on each day, but maybe not. You really do need to keep off of sugar during these two days. Follow your surgeon's instructions.

Chapter 7: Your Diet on Surgery Day and Beyond

If you think you can cheat on your diet now, you are wrong! You cannot cheat on your diet after your surgery or you will suffer. Your pre-op diet was for the purpose of reducing risk *during* your surgery. Your post-op diet (the first four weeks after surgery) will be for the purpose of reducing the risk of *post-op complications*.

Your surgeon is not being overly cautious when he tells you to continue to consume clear liquids. It is important that you continue to follow the prescribed diet very closely.

If you cheat on your diet, you may cause a very serious gastric leak, where food gets through the staple line, out of your digestive system and into your abdominal area. If that happens early, the surgeon will get back in there and flush you out. If that happens later, it will progress to an infection that can become life-threatening.

Cheating could also cause constipation, diarrhea, or even bowel obstruction. Just don't do it! Stay the course and you will be able to gradually add back foods that you love without creating problems (and possibly another surgery) for yourself.

You will be in pain after your surgery, so it will be normal for you to be irritable during this time and to wonder whether or not you should have had the surgery. But this too will pass!

Surgery Day – Nothing by Mouth

You will probably be thirsty after your operation, but you won't be allowed to drink anything until the day after your operation. The breathing tube that was put down your throat would make drinking unpleasant anyway. Your surgeon may allow mouth swabs or an occasional cup of ice.

Day One – Drink Test and Discharge Day

A radiologist will give you a swallow test that will test for major leaks in your stomach area before you will be allowed by the surgeon to have water to drink. You should only have a small amount of anything on this day.

No carbonated drinks or drinks with caffeine will be allowed on this day. Caffeine creates a diuretic effect, which is a major reason patients who cheat and drink something with caffeine are readmitted for dehydration!

Don't accept drinks or food from well-meaning family or friends that are off of the list of allowed drinks or food. Follow the doctor's orders. There is a good reason for not consuming whatever he tells you not to consume!

You will likely just be thirsty on this day, but if you do want something other than water, your choices will be as follows:

- Sugar-free gelatin
- Strained cream soup
- Milk
- Unsweetened juice
- Broth

Days Two and Three – On Your Own

Your spouse may be back at work. You will likely need to get whatever you consume on your own unless you have children or unemployed friends lined up to help you after you get home.

What you are allowed to eat on these two days is up to your surgeon. You may still be on the liquid diet for the remainder of the week. Alternatively, you may be allowed to advance to pureed food at some point during your first week following surgery.

If you can have pureed food, it cannot have lumps in it. The food allowed will likely include the following items:

- Soft fruit
- Yogurt
- Fish
- Beans
- Lean ground meat

Liquids allowed will likely include the following:

- Broth
- Juice
- Fat-free milk
- Water

Your body is used to getting a lot of its fluids from food, but it won't get all that it needs from food now. You need to drink a lot of fluids from now on. Check your sugar levels if you are diabetic. Your diabetes meds have likely been reduced now as part of the discharge plan.

Week One – Clear Liquids Only

As previously stated, you won't likely have much desire to eat food right after you have your surgery because the hunger hormone (ghrelin) won't exist within you. That is because the area of the stomach where most of that hormone was manufactured has been removed. You may or may not be off of the clear liquid diet by days two and three.

You cannot have caffeine, sugar, sweet beverages or carbonated beverages at this stage, so your clear-liquid options that you can consume during this early time period consisting of the following:

- Sugar-free drinks (flat or otherwise has no carbonation)

- Sugar-free popsicles

- Decaffeinated coffee

- Decaffeinated tea

- Jell-O

- Broth

- Water

Week Two – Liquid Diet with Protein

You may actually be a little hungry by now, but it will likely be a week that involves tasty protein shakes. Yum! Hopefully, you pre-made, tested, tweaked, and froze a bunch of different flavors of shakes and smoothies before your surgery. Hopefully, the family has stayed out of them too!

Eat whatever the surgeon tells you to eat, but your diet will likely include the following choices:

- Protein powder mixed with a clear liquid that is sugar-free and non-carbonated

- Cream soups thinned out with water and containing no chunks in it

- Soups with soft noodles

- Sugar-free sorbet

- Sugar-free pudding

- Non-fat yogurt

- Sugar-free and very watery hot oatmeal

- Diluted, no sugar added juice

- Thinned applesauce with no sugar added

Week Three – Soft Pureed Food

This will likely be a tough week for you. You will be able to add some normal food to your diet, though pureed, some of it will likely make you sick.

Some food may taste different to you now. Some food may not be tolerated well after your surgery, such as dairy. If you introduce food one by one, you will be able to identify food that you have trouble with so as to avoid it for a while.

You will also document what each offending food did to you. Did it cause gas, upset your stomach, cause diarrhea? If you premade shakes, know what you put into the shakes so that you can document the ingredients from which one or more may not yet agree with your new digestive system.

Continue to limit sugar and fat. This week you have three goals you need to reach, which are:

- Consume 60 grams of protein every day (more if you are a man).
- Eat your food slowly.
- Introduce new food one at a time, not during the same meal.

During this week, you need to AVOID the following items:

- Fibrous vegetables such as broccoli, celery, asparagus and raw leafy greens

- Starchy foods like pasta, rice, and bread

- Sugar – Note: Even your protein smoothies and shakes can have too much sugar in the form of fructose, so you may need to consume those extra fruity drinks in smaller doses than the other smoothies and shakes during this stage.

Food choices for this week include the following items:

- One protein shake or smoothie per day, which can be blended with yogurt or non-fat milk or even cottage cheese

- Almond milk in shakes

- Coconut milk in shakes

- Hummus

- Low-fat cottage cheese

- Soft cheeses in limited amount (high in fat)

- Soft (soggy) cereal

- Soft steamed or boiled vegetables

- Ground beef mixed with stock to keep it soft

- Ground chicken mixed with stock to keep it soft

- Soups

- Scrambled eggs (good source of protein)

- Canned tuna mixed with low-fat mayonnaise (good source of protein)

- Canned salmon mixed with low-fat mayonnaise (good source of protein)

- Mashed fruit that has not had sugar added to it. Bananas are great

- Mashed avocados

Week Four – Introduce Real Food

While you do not have to eat pureed food this week, you still need to eat softer versions of the various food options and you need to continue to chew your food well.

Your stomach is still sensitive. You need to AVOID the following food items:

- Sodas
- Sugary drinks
- Candy
- Dessert
- Fried foods
- Nuts
- High-carbohydrate food such as pasta, bread, pizza
- Whole milk
- Whole milk dairy foods

This week's menu can contain food such as the following:

- Protein shakes daily
- Beef and chicken introduced slowly and chewed thoroughly
- Fish of any kind
- Vegetables, soft
- Sweet potatoes
- Mashed potatoes
- Baked potatoes
- Cereal
- Caffeine, a limited amount can be introduced

If your surgeon approves of you having *snacks* between meals, they may include foods such as the following:

- Fresh fruit
- One-quarter of a baked sweet potato
- One-quarter cup of oatmeal
- One hard-boiled egg
- Hummus on rice crackers
- Hummus with boiled baby carrots

Week Five to Month Three

Continue to introduce food one by one and notate how well you take each one. Eating something you don't tolerate well will give you constipation, upset stomach, or diarrhea.

You will still eat things like cooked vegetables, canned or soft fruit, ground meat and finely diced meat. Do NOT eat much in the way of solid, hard food yet. You must wait until the doctor clears you for those kinds of foods.

Guidelines

- Eat three meals daily, still concentrating on protein intake.

- Drink lots of fluids throughout every day, but stop drinking 30 minutes before each meal.

- Try not to snack unless you have something nutritious, such as fruit, veggies or maybe a few nuts.

- Remember to take your vitamins.

- Make sure you get around 60 grams of protein (get a little more if you are a man), drinking a protein shake every day in addition to the small amount of food you are eating.

- Make a habit of doing some sort of exercise every day.

- As always, avoid sodas, although you can have a little bit of caffeine (tea, coffee) now.

- Be prepared for bad days so that you can cope.

- Find yourself an accountability partner in a support group or somewhere that you can call.

Month Three to Month Six and Beyond

You should have lost a very noticeable amount of weight by now and are very glad you had the surgery.

Your surgeon will likely approve you for solid foods now. You will feel full very fast now when you eat them. Chew them well. Eat slowly.

You need to take it slowly because crunchy and/or spicy food may be difficult to tolerate at first. As before, you need to introduce one solid food at a time and see how well your system handles it. Document any problems, as always.

You should have a dietician that you meet with regularly by now. They will help you strategize blending your diet with those of your family's and give you grocery shopping tips and tips for getting through holiday meals, etc.

General Tips

To help you in your journey, here are six useful tips:

- Choose foods that contain a lot of nutrients. For example, fish and fruit contain lots of nutrients, but bread does not have much value.

- Don't drink your calories. Calorie-filled drinks usually contain a lot of sugar and they don't fill you up.

- Create a plan to deal with emotional days when you will be tempted to use food to comfort yourself with.

- Take your time eating your food, chewing everything very thoroughly.

- When you eat out, eat half a portion size. You may be able to split a meal with somebody else who then orders a side dish or two to complete their meal. Alternatively, you could get a box and take half of your meal home with you or see whether or not the restaurant would give you a discount for ordering half a meal.

- Buy yourself a reusable 64-ounce bottle that you can carry with you. Fill it with water and drink all of the water every day, remembering to not drink fluids with meals.

  The reason you should not drink with your meals is that your stomach doesn't hold nearly as much as it did before your surgery, so you need to utilize the space for meals. You also don't want to run the risk of stretching out your stomach pouch. It is possible to stretch it out, accommodating more food, which defeats the purpose of getting the pouch size cut via the sleeve gastrectomy.

Chapter 8: Vitamins and Minerals

Whatever type of gastric surgery you have had, you will need to take vitamins and supplements for the rest of your life. Bypass patients need the most, followed by sleeve patients and then lab band patients.

Even people who have not had gastric surgery should take vitamins and supplements because our food is lacking the nutrition that it used to have. Additionally, people seldom make good food choices.

None of us are getting the nutrition we need in the United States unless we take vitamins and supplements. But for the gastric patient, it is no longer physically possible to take in sufficient nutrients just from food, even if the patient ate only quality food.

A gastric sleeve patient will typically need to take a multivitamin and minerals, iron, calcium citrate, vitamin B12, and protein supplements, although taking more vitamins would be even better. Let's look at each one of these supplements.

Multivitamin and minerals

You will need a chewable multivitamin the first month following your surgery, possibly taking one in the morning and one at night. Bariatric Advantage and Bariatric Fusion are good ones for bariatric patients. Centrum Adult Daily Chewable is an option for the non-bariatric consumer, and it can be found at common local pharmacies such as Walgreens.

Iron

Your surgeon may recommend that you take iron. If he does, he'll tell you to take it on an empty stomach. Do not buy the typical ferrous sulfate because your body will not absorb it after your surgery. What you need is Ferrous Fumarate 29mg. Do not take it when you take your Calcium Citrate, however.

Calcium Citrate

You will start to take this supplement one month after your surgery. You can get it in chewable form or in liquid form. Take this supplement three times daily for a total of between 1500 and 2000 mg. Spread your doses apart by at least one hour in between doses.

As stated in the iron paragraph above, you should not take Calcium Citrate at the same time that you take the iron. In fact, you need to separate taking the Calcium Citrate from when you take both your multivitamin and iron supplements by at least two hours.

Vitamin B12

You typically take this vitamin one time per week at a dosage of between 5000 and 7500 mg. You can get it sublingually (under your tongue), by injection, or by nasal spray. Do not take this in pill form after your surgery.

Protein supplements

You need to have at least 60 mg of protein daily. In supplement form, surgeons prefer that you buy a bariatric-specific protein supplement, such as Bariatric Advantage, Unjury, or Bariatric Fusion, instead of the kind you find at common retailers.

Of course, you will use a lot of protein powder in smoothies and shakes that you make.

There are also a few commercially-made brands that are low enough in sugar to suffice, although you really need to stay away from any with sugar if you can help it. They are as follows:

- MET-Rx Protein Plus – This drink delivers 51 grams of protein and only two grams of sugar within each 260-calorie drink.

- Nature's Best Zero Carb Isopure – This drink delivers up to 40 grams of protein and no carbs within each 160-calorie drink.

- CytoSport Monster Milk – This drink delivers 45 grams of protein and **no sugar** within each drink. It also contains five grams of dietary fiber in every drink.

- Muscle Milk Pro – This drink delivers 40 grams of protein and two grams of sugar in each lactose-free and gluten-free drink. This brand can be found more easily than the others can, and can even be found in gas stations and convenience stores.

- Shakeology – This drink delivers 17 grams of protein and six grams of sugar in each drink, which makes it not the best choice. However, it does give you the added benefit of 70 vitamins, minerals, probiotics, prebiotics, fiber, digestive enzymes, antioxidants, and phytonutrients.

- Pure Protein Shakes – This drink delivers between 23 and 35 grams of protein, depending on the size and flavor, in each drink while including just one gram of sugar and no aspartame. Each drink also gives you three grams of fiber, some calcium, and other benefits.

Chapter 9: Stomach Stretching after Surgery

Besides getting rid of most of the hunger hormone, the other purpose of the surgery is to shrink the stomach size so as to feel full faster. Whether or not the stomach could stretch out, enabling the weight to come back on, is one of the top questions that people ask about gastric sleeve surgery. After all, a person goes through money, pain, trouble and a small risk of complications for the purpose of losing weight and keeping the weight off.

It is possible to stretch the smaller stomach out, but whether or not the stomach stretches back out and the weight returns is up to the patient. The surgery makes the stomach smaller and gets rid of much of the hunger hormones, so the patient is given a good advantage over other people when it comes to keeping the weight off.

This advantage should enable success for the remainder of the patient's life, however, it is possible to mess this up. The patient must actively keep their stomach small.

The other factor affecting the weight gain part of the equation, of course, is whether or not the patient also maintains the new diet and exercise lifestyle. Consuming just sugary and fat food, even in a small stomach, will pack the pounds back on. The surgery is a tool, not a quick fix. The patient must work at his weight loss goal for the rest of his or her life.

Know how hunger and fullness signals get messed up.

Let's take a closer look at how the stomach works. The walls of your stomach contain folds of tissue that expand and contract in response to the food that enters and leaves the stomach. When the stomach expands far enough, a signal goes to your brain that tells it you have eaten enough food. Your stomach is full.

Acid starts to break down the food as soon as it enters. The stomach walls contract to push the food on down to your intestines for further digestion of the food.

If you overeat and stretch the walls too often, the stomach tells the brain that it is full later than it should. It also tells the brain that it is hungry when it still contains food. This broken signal system causes you to eat more food on a regular basis, which is what makes losing weight difficult for people in the first place.

Keep yourself on track using several tricks.

An occasional large meal such as one at Thanksgiving, won't mess up the signals, however, habitual overeating will permanently stretch out your stomach and mess up the signals.

Here are some tips for keeping your stomach small after surgery:

- You already limit the sugar in your diet, which is likely hard for you. Give yourself a reward every week, but make the reward a small sweet treat instead of a large meal, even if it would have been a healthy large meal.

- Don't drink when you eat. Drink your fluids one or two hours before or after you eat so that the fluids don't increase the amount of gas in your system or take up stomach space you need for the small amount of food you will eat.

- After an occasional large meal, make sure that your next meal is small and that you don't make those large ones a habit.

- If you stay hungry, eat small amounts of healthy snacks between your small meals. Almonds make a satisfying and healthy snack.

- Get a good recipe book that is geared for gastric sleeve patients.

- Get back on track, even if you overeat for up to a week. Don't get discouraged. If you have ongoing trouble keeping the amount of food you eat under control, call your surgeon.

- Ask for helpful information from people in the online forums. You are anonymous there anyway.

Take control of the portion size when others try to control it.

The restaurants often serve portion sizes that are already enough for two smallish adults. They make more money by doing that. When you eat at a restaurant or in some other situation, such as at somebody's home, where somebody else tries to control your portion size, you must take control of how much food you eat during that meal.

In those restaurant situations, you can take control of your portion size (and save a lot of money over time) the following ways:

- Get a box to take the other half of your meal home to eat later.

- Split the meal with somebody you are eating out with.

- Request a lunch size.

- Order a couple of side dishes or an appetizer instead of a full meal.

At somebody's home, tell the person who is putting food on your plate how much you want.

The bottom line is that you must actively keep your stomach small.

Conclusion

Thank you again for downloading this book!

I hope this book was able to answer many questions that you may have had about the gastric sleeve procedure and that it helped those of you who have not yet had a sleeve gastrectomy to be confident in your choice to have the surgery and to know what to do before and after you have it.

Hopefully, those of you who have already gone through the procedure realize how important it is to not cheat on your diet, and you hopefully also have a good understanding of how to succeed in keeping the weight off once you are out of the danger zone.

If you have not yet had your surgery and you are confident in your decision to have it, the next step is to follow the steps outlined in Chapter Three. The surgeon you choose is an especially important factor in reducing the risk of having complications during and as a result of the surgery.

After your surgery, you need to stay on the diet and follow all of your doctor's instructions because your food choices during the recovery time directly affect the risk factor for having complications that could become life-threatening. That will not the time to cheat!

Going forward after the recovery period, you must fight your urges to eat sweets, fattening food or to overeat. You've been through a lot. Now the hard work begins. It is so worth it, though.

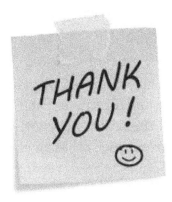

Finally, if you enjoyed this book, then I'd like to ask you for a favor. Would you be kind enough to leave a review for this book on Amazon? It would be greatly appreciated!

Click here to leave a review for this book on Amazon!

Thank you and good luck!

Check Out My Other Books

Below you'll find some of my other popular books that are popular on Amazon and Kindle as well. Simply click on the links below to check them out. Alternatively, you can visit my author page on Amazon to see other work done by me.

CrossFit: Barbell and Dumbbell Exercises for Body Strength

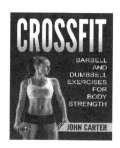

Mediterranean Diet: Step By Step Guide And Proven Recipes For Smart Eating And Weight Loss

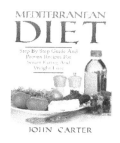

Weight Watchers: Smart Points Cookbook - Step By Step Guide And Proven Recipes For Effective Weight Loss

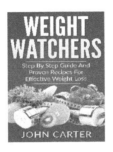

Bodybuilding: Beginners Handbook - Proven Step By Step Guide To Get The Body You Always Dreamed About

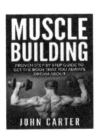

South Beach Diet: Lose Weight and Get Healthy the South Beach Way

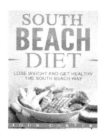

Blood Pressure: Step By Step Guide And Proven Recipes To Lower Your Blood Pressure Without Any Medication

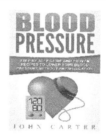

Ketogenic Diet: Step By Step Guide And 70+ Low Carb, Proven Recipes For Rapid Weight Loss

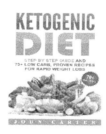

<u>Meal Prep: 65+ Meal Prep Recipes Cookbook –
Step By Step Meal Prepping Guide For Rapid
Weight Loss</u>

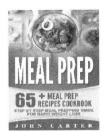

If the links do not work, for whatever reason, you can simply search for these titles on the Amazon website to find them.